Mastering Luc...

Techniques, Tips, and the Science of Controlling Your Dreams

Clara Müller

Introduction to Lucid Dreaming

Lucid dreaming is the practice of becoming aware that you are dreaming, allowing you to control and manipulate the dream as it unfolds. For many, lucid dreaming offers the opportunity to explore limitless possibilities within a self-created, virtual reality. But it is more than just a playground for the mind—it is also a powerful tool for self-discovery, problem-solving, and even emotional healing.

History of Lucid Dreaming

The concept of lucid dreaming has been referenced throughout human history. The Ancient Egyptians were among the first cultures to document dreams in a symbolic way, often interpreting them as divine messages. Similarly, in Tibetan Buddhism, the practice of dream yoga is an ancient spiritual technique in which practitioners train themselves to maintain awareness during dreams. The purpose of dream yoga is to use dreams as a vehicle for enlightenment by recognizing the dreamlike nature of all experiences, both waking and dreaming.

In Western psychology, lucid dreaming gained prominence in the early 20th century when Dutch psychiatrist Frederik van Eeden coined the term "lucid dreaming" to describe the phenomenon of dreamers becoming conscious within their dreams. However, it wasn't until the 1970s, when Dr. Stephen LaBerge at Stanford University conducted pioneering studies on lucid dreaming, that the phenomenon gained scientific validation.

Why Learn Lucid Dreaming?
Lucid dreaming is not just a curiosity or a means of escape; it offers numerous benefits in various aspects of life. Whether you're interested in enhancing your creativity, overcoming fears, practicing new skills, or simply enjoying the thrill of a fully immersive dream experience, lucid dreaming can help. Here are some key reasons why learning this skill is worth your time:

- **Personal Empowerment:** In lucid dreams, you have the opportunity to take control of situations, overcome challenges, and reshape outcomes— experiences that can improve your confidence in waking life.

- **Confronting Fears:** If you suffer from recurring nightmares, lucid dreaming gives you the ability to alter the course of frightening scenarios, which can lead to a greater sense of mastery over your subconscious mind.

- **Exploring the Depths of Your Mind:** Lucid dreams provide access to the deeper layers of your mind, allowing you to explore forgotten memories, emotional blockages, or creative insights that might be hidden from your conscious mind.

- **Enhanced Creativity and Problem-Solving:** Many artists, writers, and inventors have used lucid dreams as a space to explore ideas without the constraints of reality.

Lucid dreaming encourages lateral thinking, which can result in unexpected solutions to problems.

By the end of this book, you'll not only understand how to achieve lucid dreams but also how to maximize their potential for personal growth and enjoyment.

The Science Behind Dreams

To appreciate lucid dreaming fully, it helps to understand how dreaming works and the biological processes behind it. Dreams occur during specific stages of sleep, and lucid dreaming is most often associated with REM (Rapid Eye Movement) sleep, a phase characterized by vivid imagery and heightened brain activity.

The Sleep Cycle Explained

Sleep is divided into two primary types: Non-REM (NREM) and REM sleep. These types alternate in cycles that last around 90 minutes throughout the night. Here's a breakdown of the stages:

1. **Stage 1 (NREM):** This is the transition from wakefulness to sleep. During this brief phase, your brain waves slow down, and you might experience the sensation of drifting or falling. Stage 1 sleep is light and easily disturbed.

2. **Stage 2 (NREM)**: As you progress into deeper sleep, your heart rate slows, body temperature drops, and your brain begins producing rhythmic bursts of activity known as sleep spindles. Stage 2 is still a lighter phase of sleep but is crucial for preparing your body for deeper rest.

3. **Stage 3 (NREM)**: Also called slow-wave sleep or deep sleep, this phase is where your body repairs itself. Growth hormone is released, tissues are repaired, and the immune system is strengthened. While dreaming can occur in this stage, it is less vivid and memorable than in REM sleep.

4. **REM Sleep**: After passing through the NREM stages, you enter REM sleep. This is where the majority of vivid, story-like dreams happen. Your brain becomes more active, almost mirroring the activity seen during wakefulness, while your muscles become temporarily paralyzed (a condition called atonia) to prevent you from acting out your dreams.

The Role of REM Sleep in Lucid Dreaming
Lucid dreaming almost exclusively occurs during REM sleep because it's the stage in which the brain is most active and capable of producing the surreal, yet highly detailed, dream environments. During REM, the prefrontal cortex—the part of your brain responsible for decision-making and self-awareness—often remains dormant, which is why we typically don't question the bizarre logic of dreams.

However, in lucid dreams, this area of the brain "wakes up," allowing the dreamer to recognize the dream state and take control.

Scientific Research on Lucid Dreaming

Dr. Stephen LaBerge conducted the first scientific experiments proving that lucid dreaming was real. In one of his most famous experiments, he trained subjects to signal that they had become lucid in their dreams by moving their eyes in predetermined patterns (left-right-left-right) while asleep. Because eye movements are not subject to the paralysis that affects other muscles during REM sleep, this gave researchers direct evidence that the dreamers were consciously aware within their dreams. Lucid dreaming research continues today, with studies investigating how it can be used for therapeutic purposes, such as helping people overcome nightmares or manage conditions like PTSD.

What Happens in the Brain During Lucid Dreams?

When you become lucid, different regions of the brain interact in a unique way. During regular dreaming, the brain's amygdala (responsible for emotions and memories) is highly active, while the prefrontal cortex (responsible for logical thinking) is less active. In a lucid dream, however, the prefrontal cortex reactivates, allowing the dreamer to gain insight into their dream state. This increased awareness allows for the possibility of control and manipulation of the dream narrative.

Benefits of Lucid Dreaming

Lucid dreaming offers a wide array of benefits that go beyond just having fun in your dreams. The practice of becoming aware and intentional in your dreams can translate to improved skills, emotional healing, and enhanced creativity in waking life.

1. Overcoming Nightmares

For those who suffer from frequent nightmares, whether related to stress, anxiety, or trauma, lucid dreaming can be a therapeutic tool. The ability to recognize that you're in a nightmare provides an opportunity to change the narrative. For instance, instead of being chased by a monster, you can stop, turn around, and ask the monster what it represents. Many lucid dreamers report that once they confront a fear in a dream, it either dissipates or transforms into something less threatening.

Lucid dreaming therapy has been particularly effective for people dealing with Post-Traumatic Stress Disorder (PTSD). In cases where nightmares are linked to trauma, lucid dreaming allows the dreamer to take back control, reducing the emotional impact of the nightmares over time.

2. Enhancing Creativity

Because the dream world operates free from the constraints of logic and physics, it is a fertile ground for creative exploration. Lucid dreaming can allow you to engage with ideas and scenarios that would be impossible or difficult to conceive while awake.

Many artists, musicians, writers, and inventors have used dreams to enhance their creativity. For example:

- Paul McCartney dreamed the melody for "Yesterday," one of The Beatles' most famous songs.

- Salvador Dalí, the surrealist painter, frequently referenced his dreams and lucid states as a source of inspiration for his bizarre, dreamlike paintings.

Lucid dreaming allows you to intentionally engage with your creative process. For example, you can enter a dream with the intention of exploring new artistic ideas or solving creative blocks. You can visualize entire works of art or music compositions and experience them in real time within the dream. By practicing this, you're tapping into the subconscious, which is often the birthplace of original and unexpected ideas.

3. Problem-Solving and Skill Development

Many lucid dreamers report using their dreams as a way to work through complex problems or practice new skills. This might involve imagining yourself in a difficult work situation and trying out different strategies for solving it. Studies have shown that people who practice motor skills in their dreams (such as playing an instrument or performing a sports technique) can actually improve their performance in waking life.

The brain treats lucid dreaming as a form of mental rehearsal, engaging the same neural pathways as if you were awake and practicing.

For example:

- Athletes can use lucid dreaming to mentally rehearse difficult moves or visualize game strategies.

- Students can use it to review information or mentally practice public speaking.

- Professionals can imagine challenging workplace scenarios and mentally rehearse presentations, interviews, or negotiations.

4. Emotional Healing and Self-Reflection
Because lucid dreams offer a direct line to your subconscious, they provide a unique opportunity for self-exploration and emotional healing. You can use lucid dreaming to explore unresolved emotions, work through interpersonal conflicts, or confront buried memories in a safe and controlled environment. For instance, if you are holding onto guilt, regret, or resentment, you can intentionally seek out the person or situation in your dream and work through it.
The therapeutic potential of lucid dreaming is vast.

Since your emotions are heightened in dreams, the catharsis experienced in a lucid dream can carry over into waking life, helping you process difficult feelings and experiences. Some people use lucid dreaming to reconnect with loved ones who have passed away, finding closure in conversations that couldn't happen in real life.

5. Spiritual Growth and Mystical Experiences
For those interested in spirituality, lucid dreaming offers a profound means of exploration. Many spiritual traditions, from Tibetan Buddhism to Shamanic practices, emphasize dreamwork as a tool for enlightenment or self-realization. Lucid dreams can be used for exploring higher states of consciousness, seeking guidance from spiritual figures, or experiencing a connection to the universe in ways that transcend ordinary life.

Lucid dreaming can provide a deeply meditative experience where dreamers feel a sense of unity, transcendence, or spiritual insight. Some use it for meditation or to explore philosophical questions, such as the nature of reality and consciousness itself.

Preparing Your Mind for Lucidity

Becoming a proficient lucid dreamer is not something that happens overnight. It requires preparation, mental conditioning, and the development of certain habits. There are several key practices that can help prime your mind for lucidity.

1. Mindfulness in Daily Life

One of the most effective ways to train your mind for lucid dreaming is through the practice of mindfulness. Mindfulness means being fully aware of the present moment, paying attention to your thoughts, surroundings, and sensations without judgment. In your waking life, by training your mind to stay aware and present, you strengthen the mental muscles needed to become aware during a dream.

Here's how mindfulness can be incorporated into your daily routine:

- **Body Scan Meditation:** This practice involves mentally scanning your body from head to toe, focusing on each part and becoming aware of any sensations. By doing this regularly, you improve your capacity for self-awareness, which can carry over into your dream state.

- **Active Observation:** Throughout the day, take time to observe the small details around you— whether it's the texture of a wall, the color of the sky, or the sound of footsteps. Ask yourself: "Am I dreaming?"

This habit of questioning reality will eventually become second nature, making it easier to perform the same mental check when you're dreaming.

2. Reality Testing

Reality testing is a critical component of preparing for lucid dreaming. It involves regularly questioning whether you are awake or dreaming. This habit conditions your mind to do the same within a dream. To make reality checks effective, you must perform them frequently and with genuine curiosity.

Here are some common reality tests:

- **Hand Check:** Look at your hands. In dreams, hands often appear distorted, with extra fingers or strange textures. If your hands look odd, you're likely dreaming.

- **Text Test:** In a dream, text often shifts, changes, or becomes unreadable when you look away and then back. Find a piece of text in your environment, glance away, and then look back to see if it changes.

- **Nose Pinch Test:** Pinch your nose shut and try to breathe through it. If you can still breathe, you're in a dream.

Make reality testing a habit by doing it multiple times a day.

It's especially effective to perform a reality check whenever something strange or out of the ordinary happens, as that's a likely time for your brain to cue in on the dream state.

3. Dream Journaling
Keeping a dream journal is one of the most powerful tools for becoming a lucid dreamer. By writing down your dreams, you strengthen your dream recall, making it easier to spot patterns, recurring symbols, and personal "dream signs" that can trigger lucidity.
Here's how to effectively keep a dream journal:

- **Keep it Close:** Keep your journal and a pen next to your bed. As soon as you wake up, write down everything you can remember from your dreams, no matter how fragmented or trivial. The sooner you record the details, the more likely you are to remember them accurately.

- **Focus on Details:** Try to capture not just the events of the dream, but also the emotions, sensations, and oddities. These often provide clues to future lucid dreams.

- **Analyze Patterns:** After a week or two of journaling, review your entries. Look for recurring themes, people, places, or objects. These are your personal dream signs, and recognizing them can help you realize you're dreaming.

4. Intention Setting Before Sleep

Another key preparation is setting a clear intention before sleep. Intention setting is a form of mental conditioning where you remind yourself that you will become lucid in your dreams. You can do this by repeating a simple mantra before you fall asleep, such as: "Tonight, I will realize I'm dreaming." Repeating this mantra several times helps to solidify the idea in your subconscious, increasing the likelihood that you will recognize the dream state when it happens.

This technique, called Mnemonic Induction of Lucid Dreams (MILD), was popularized by Stephen LaBerge and remains one of the most reliable methods for inducing lucid dreams.

5. Sleep Environment Optimization

The quality of your sleep environment plays a critical role in your ability to achieve lucid dreams. A comfortable, peaceful sleep environment encourages deep, restorative sleep and more vivid REM periods.

Here's how to optimize your environment for lucid dreaming:

- **Eliminate Distractions**: Make sure your bedroom is free from disruptive sounds, harsh lights, and uncomfortable temperatures. Use earplugs, white noise machines, or blackout curtains if necessary.

- **Comfortable Bedding:** A comfortable mattress and pillows are essential for restful sleep.

If you're frequently waking up due to discomfort, it will be harder to enter the deep sleep needed for vivid dreams.

- **Sleep Schedule:** Stick to a regular sleep schedule. Going to bed and waking up at the same time every day helps regulate your sleep cycles, particularly your REM cycles, which are critical for lucid dreaming.

6. Supplements and Sleep Aids

There are some natural supplements known to enhance dream vividness and REM activity, potentially aiding lucid dreaming.

While these are not necessary, some lucid dreamers find them helpful:

- **Vitamin B6:** This vitamin has been shown in studies to improve dream vividness and recall. Taking it before bed may help.

- **Choline and Galantamine:** These supplements work by increasing acetylcholine levels in the brain, a neurotransmitter involved in memory and REM sleep. However, they should be used with caution and ideally under guidance, as they can disrupt normal sleep patterns if misused.

With your mind properly prepared, you will be ready to explore the world of lucid dreaming.

The next chapters will delve into the specific techniques for inducing and maintaining lucid dreams, as well as how to gain full control once inside the dream world.

The Foundation of Lucid Dreaming

Reality checks are the backbone of any successful lucid dreaming practice. They train your mind to question whether you are awake or dreaming. The more often you perform reality checks during waking life, the more likely you are to perform one in a dream, which can trigger lucidity.

Why Reality Checks Work
In dreams, we often fail to question the strange or illogical things happening around us because our logical thinking is suppressed. The dream feels real, even if something absurd is happening, like flying or interacting with impossible creatures. By making reality checks a habit in waking life, you train your brain to bring this same critical thinking into the dream state, allowing you to become aware that you're dreaming.
Common Reality Checks.
Here are some of the most reliable reality checks, each of which exploits the inherent oddities of dream logic:

1. **Hand Check:** Look at your hands. In dreams, your hands may appear distorted—extra fingers, blurred lines, or strange textures. This is because fine details like fingers are often poorly rendered in dreams.

Focus on your hands for a few seconds; if they appear odd, you are likely dreaming.

- o *How to practice:* Throughout the day, take a moment to examine your hands closely. Ask yourself, "Am I dreaming?" while focusing on their appearance.

2. **Text Check:** In the dream world, text often changes when you look away and then look back at it. Signs, books, or even digital clocks are rarely stable in dreams.

- o *How to practice:* Look at a piece of text, glance away, and then quickly glance back. If the text has changed or is unreadable, it's a strong indicator that you're in a dream.

3. **Nose Pinch Test:** One of the simplest and most effective reality checks is to pinch your nose shut and try to breathe through it. In a dream, even with your nose pinched, you will still be able to breathe, because your brain isn't constrained by physical laws.

- o *How to practice:* Periodically pinch your nose and attempt to breathe through it. If you can breathe, you're dreaming.

4. **Mirror Test:** Mirrors are notoriously unreliable in dreams. Your reflection might look blurry, distorted, or even fail to appear entirely.

- *How to practice:* Whenever you pass a mirror, pause and examine your reflection. If anything appears strange, it's a clue that you're in a dream.

5. **Finger-Through-Palm:** In dreams, physical boundaries are often flexible. Try pushing your index finger through the palm of your opposite hand. In a dream, your finger will often pass through without resistance.

   - *How to practice:* Every time you perform this check, mentally ask, "Am I dreaming?" Imagine your finger passing through your palm to help reinforce the idea.

How Often Should You Perform Reality Checks?

To make reality checks a habit, aim to perform them at least 10–15 times per day. Key times to do reality checks are:

- Whenever something unusual or odd happens (e.g., a strange coincidence).

- Whenever you enter a new environment (e.g., walking into a new room).

- When you experience strong emotions, since heightened emotions often occur in dreams.

- Right before going to sleep, to solidify the habit in your mind.

The more often you perform reality checks, the more likely you are to incorporate them into your dreams, which is the key to achieving lucidity.
Combining Reality Checks with Intention Setting
For maximum effectiveness, combine reality checks with intention setting (discussed in Chapter 4). For example, when you perform a reality check, say to yourself, "Tonight, I will become lucid in my dream." This reinforces both habits and increases your chances of realizing you're dreaming once you're in the dream state.

The Power of Dream Journaling

Dream journaling is a crucial technique for anyone serious about lucid dreaming. Not only does it help with dream recall, but it also allows you to identify recurring dream signs, themes, and symbols that can trigger lucidity.

Why Dream Journaling is Essential
One of the biggest obstacles to lucid dreaming is poor dream recall. If you can't remember your dreams, it becomes much harder to become lucid within them. Keeping a dream journal improves your dream recall by training your brain to pay closer attention to dreams. The more you record your dreams, the more detailed and vivid your recollection will become over time.
How to Keep a Dream Journal:

1. **Record Dreams Immediately:** Keep your dream journal and a pen next to your bed so you can write down your dreams as soon as you wake up.

The longer you wait, the more details will fade. If you wake up in the middle of the night, jot down key details before falling back asleep.

2. **Focus on Details:** Write down everything you remember, no matter how trivial it seems—colors, locations, people, emotions, and even fragmented images. The act of writing reinforces memory and will help you recognize patterns later.

3. **Use Voice Recording:** If writing feels cumbersome right after waking up, consider using a voice recorder. Dictate your dreams while the memory is fresh, and transcribe them later into your journal.

4. **Look for Dream Signs**: After a few weeks of journaling, review your entries and look for recurring themes, symbols, or situations. These are your dream signs—unique elements that can signal to you that you're dreaming. Common dream signs include flying, being chased, interacting with certain people, or visiting specific locations. These are your cues to become lucid.

5. **Reflect on Emotions:** Note how you felt during the dream. Emotional intensity is often a key factor in dreams, and understanding these emotions can help you in future dream interpretation and lucidity.

Dream Journaling Tips

- **Stay Consistent:** Try to record your dreams daily, even if you don't remember much. This practice will improve your recall over time.

- **Illustrate:** If you're a visual person, sketch out key elements of your dream. This can be especially helpful for recalling dream landscapes or symbolic objects.

- **Dream Triggers:** Make a note of any "odd" or out-of-place events that occur in your dreams. These can become triggers for reality checks in future dreams.

How Dream Journaling Leads to Lucidity
By reviewing your journal regularly, you'll start to see patterns that can serve as dream signs. These recurring elements act as cues that you can use to realize you're dreaming. For instance, if you often dream of being on a beach, and you find yourself on a beach in a dream, you can perform a reality check, recognize you're dreaming, and become lucid.
In addition to aiding in lucidity, dream journaling can be a powerful tool for personal growth. Dreams often provide insights into your subconscious mind, revealing thoughts and feelings that you might not be fully aware of in your waking life.

WILD and DILD: The Two Key Techniques

Lucid dreaming can be achieved through various techniques, but two of the most effective and widely practiced are Wake-Induced Lucid Dreaming (WILD) and Dream-Induced Lucid Dreaming (DILD). Each method has its unique approach and challenges.

Dream-Induced Lucid Dreaming (DILD)

DILD is when you become lucid while already inside a dream, usually triggered by recognizing something unusual (like a dream sign) or performing a reality check. DILD is considered more natural and is often the first method people experience when they have spontaneous lucid dreams.

How to Induce DILD

- **Reality Checks:** As described in Chapter 5, reality checks are the primary method for inducing a DILD. By making reality checks a habit, you train yourself to question reality in a dream, which can lead to lucidity.

- **Dream Signs:** Analyzing your dream journal to identify recurring dream signs is another method to increase your chances of achieving DILD. For example, if you frequently dream of flying, you can train yourself to perform a reality check whenever you notice this sign.

- **MILD Technique:** The Mnemonic Induction of Lucid Dreams (MILD) technique, developed by

Stephen LaBerge, involves setting an intention before sleep to recognize when you are dreaming. You can combine this with reality checks and dream signs to increase the likelihood of becoming lucid.

Wake-Induced Lucid Dreaming (WILD)
WILD is a technique where you transition directly from a waking state into a lucid dream without losing consciousness. While it is a more challenging method, WILD can be extremely powerful because it allows for immediate, conscious entry into the dream world.

How to Perform WILD:

1. **Relaxation:** The first step in WILD is to relax your body completely. Lie down in a comfortable position, close your eyes, and focus on your breathing. Allow your body to enter a deep state of relaxation, but keep your mind alert.

2. **Hypnagogic Imagery:** As you start to fall asleep, you'll begin to see hypnagogic imagery—fleeting images, shapes, and scenes. These are the precursors to entering the dream state. Focus on these images without becoming too attached to them.

3. **Stay Conscious:** The challenge of WILD is maintaining awareness while your body falls asleep. As you approach sleep, you may experience sleep paralysis (a normal part of REM sleep).

Don't panic—this is a sign that you're close to entering the dream state.

4. **Enter the Dream:** As your body falls asleep, the hypnagogic imagery will gradually turn into a full dream environment. At this point, you can "step into" the dream, fully aware and in control.

Challenges with WILD
WILD can be tricky because it requires a delicate balance between staying conscious and allowing your body to fall asleep. If your mind stays too alert, you'll remain awake. If you relax too much, you'll fall asleep unconsciously. Practicing meditation or mindfulness can help develop the focus needed to master WILD.
Combining WILD with the Wake-Back-to-Bed (WBTB)

Method
Many people find success with WILD by combining it with the Wake-Back-to-Bed (WBTB) method. This involves waking up after 4-6 hours of sleep, staying awake for 10-30 minutes, and then returning to bed with the intention of entering a lucid dream. The WBTB method works because you're entering REM sleep more quickly after going back to bed, which is the most favorable time for lucid dreaming.

Mastering Sleep Cycles for Lucid Dreams

Understanding and optimizing your sleep cycles is a critical aspect of becoming a proficient lucid dreamer. Lucid dreams occur most frequently during REM sleep, so learning to work with your body's natural rhythms can significantly increase your chances of having lucid dreams.

Understanding the Sleep Cycle

The sleep cycle lasts about 90 minutes and repeats multiple times throughout the night. Each cycle consists of:

- **NREM Sleep:** Stages 1, 2, and 3 of Non-REM sleep, where your body relaxes and repairs itself. Dreams are less vivid in these stages, and you are less likely to become lucid.

- **REM Sleep:** Rapid Eye Movement sleep is where most dreaming occurs. This phase gets longer with each cycle throughout the night, meaning that your longest and most vivid dreams happen in the early morning hours.

How to Use Sleep Cycles to Induce Lucid Dreams

Because REM sleep is the most favorable stage for lucid dreaming, it's essential to time your lucid dreaming attempts to coincide with REM periods.

Here are a few techniques to help you do that:

1.   The Wake-Back-to-Bed (WBTB) Method
The WBTB method is one of the most effective ways to induce lucid dreams. Here's how it works:

- *Step 1:* Set an alarm to wake you up after 4-6 hours of sleep. This ensures that you wake up during or just after a REM period.

- *Step 2:* Stay awake for 10-30 minutes. During this time, you can meditate, read about lucid dreaming, or perform reality checks to prime your mind for lucidity.

- *Step 3:* Go back to bed with the intention of entering a lucid dream. Because you're returning to sleep directly into a REM cycle, you're more likely to enter a dream state quickly and achieve lucidity.

2.   REM Rebound Effect
The REM rebound effect occurs when you deprive yourself of REM sleep (either by staying awake longer or having interrupted sleep) and then experience a subsequent increase in REM sleep the next night. Some lucid dreamers use this effect to their advantage by intentionally limiting REM sleep for one night and then having a much longer and more vivid REM period the following night.

Tracking Your Sleep Cycles

Many modern devices, such as fitness trackers or smartphone apps, can help you track your sleep patterns. These tools monitor your sleep stages and provide data on how long you spend in each phase, allowing you to optimize your attempts at lucid dreaming. By identifying when you naturally enter REM sleep, you can tailor your techniques (like WBTB or WILD) for maximum effectiveness.

Optimizing Sleep Hygiene for Better REM Sleep

Good sleep hygiene is essential for achieving regular REM sleep and increasing your chances of lucid dreaming.

Here are a few tips to optimize your sleep:

- **Consistent Sleep Schedule:** Go to bed and wake up at the same time every day, even on weekends. This helps regulate your body's internal clock, leading to more consistent REM cycles.

- **Limit Stimulants:** Avoid caffeine, nicotine, and other stimulants in the afternoon and evening, as they can interfere with REM sleep.

- **Exercise:** Regular physical activity can improve the quality of your sleep, but try to avoid vigorous exercise too close to bedtime.

- **Relaxation Techniques:** Incorporate relaxation techniques, such as deep breathing, meditation, or reading, into your bedtime routine to reduce stress and help you transition into sleep smoothly.

By mastering your sleep cycles and creating an optimal sleep environment, you set the stage for more frequent and vivid lucid dreams.

Visualization and Meditation for Lucid Awareness

Visualization and meditation are powerful tools for developing lucid awareness, both in waking life and within dreams. These practices can train your mind to be more present, focused, and aware, which increases your chances of recognizing the dream state.
Visualization Techniques for Lucid Dreaming
Visualization involves mentally rehearsing the experience of becoming lucid. By visualizing yourself becoming aware in a dream, you reinforce the habit in your subconscious mind, making it more likely to happen when you're actually dreaming.
Here are a few effective visualization techniques:

1.   Lucid Dream Rehearsal
This technique involves visualizing a scenario in which you become lucid in a dream. Close your eyes and imagine yourself in a dream environment—perhaps a recurring dream setting from your dream journal. In your visualization, notice something odd (like a dream sign), perform a reality check, and realize that you're dreaming. Then, imagine what you would do in your lucid dream. This mental rehearsal primes your brain for the experience of becoming lucid.

o   *How to practice:* Set aside 5-10 minutes
     before bed to visualize yourself becoming
     lucid in a dream. The more vividly you can
     imagine the experience, the more effective
     this practice will be.

2.   Visualizing Desired Dream Outcomes

If there's a particular goal you want to achieve in a lucid
dream—such as flying, meeting a specific person, or
visiting a certain place—spend time visualizing that
outcome before bed. Imagine the sensations, sights, and
emotions associated with your goal. This can help guide
the direction of your lucid dreams and make it easier to
control the dream once you become lucid.

Meditation for Lucid Awareness

Meditation is another powerful tool for cultivating the
awareness needed for lucid dreaming. By training your
mind to focus and remain present, you increase your
ability to recognize when you're in a dream state.
Here are two meditation practices that are particularly
useful for lucid dreamers:

1.   Mindfulness Meditation

Mindfulness meditation involves focusing your attention
on the present moment without judgment. By practicing
mindfulness, you become more aware of your thoughts,
feelings, and surroundings, which carries over into the
dream world. When you're more mindful in waking life,
you're more likely to recognize when something is out of
place in a dream and become lucid.

o   *How to practice*: Set aside 10-15 minutes
       each day to sit in a quiet place and focus on
       your breath. Whenever your mind wanders,
       gently bring your attention back to your
       breath. Over time, this practice will enhance
       your ability to stay present and aware, both
       in waking life and in dreams.

2.   Hypnagogic Meditation

The hypnagogic state is the transition between
wakefulness and sleep, where you often experience
random thoughts, images, and sensations. Practicing
meditation during this state can help you maintain
awareness as you drift into sleep, which is particularly
useful for the WILD technique.

o   *How to practice*: As you lie in bed ready to
       fall asleep, focus on your breath and observe
       the hypnagogic imagery that appears. Try
       not to get too absorbed in the images—
       simply observe them with a calm, detached
       awareness. The goal is to remain conscious
       as your body falls asleep, allowing you to
       enter a lucid dream directly.

The Power of Combining Visualization and Meditation
Combining visualization and meditation can greatly
enhance your chances of becoming lucid. By regularly
practicing mindfulness and visualizing yourself becoming
lucid, you create strong mental habits that carry over into
your dreams.

These practices also improve your focus and mental clarity, making it easier to maintain lucidity once you achieve it.

By developing a routine that includes both visualization and meditation, you can cultivate the mental discipline needed to become a proficient lucid dreamer.

Common Lucid Dreaming Challenges and How to Overcome Them

While lucid dreaming can be an exhilarating experience, it's not without its challenges. Many people encounter obstacles along the way, whether it's difficulty maintaining lucidity, waking up too quickly, or struggling to control the dream. This chapter will explore some of the most common challenges lucid dreamers face and offer practical solutions to overcome them.

1. Difficulty Achieving Lucidity

One of the most common challenges for beginners is simply becoming lucid in the first place. It can be frustrating to practice reality checks, keep a dream journal, and set intentions, only to remain in non-lucid dreams. Here are some tips to help:

- **Be Patient:** Achieving lucidity is a skill, and like any skill, it takes time to develop. Don't get discouraged if it doesn't happen right away. Consistency is key.

- **Increase Reality Checks:** If you're struggling to become lucid, try increasing the frequency of your reality checks. Perform them during moments of heightened emotion or when you encounter strange or unexpected events in waking life, as these moments often parallel dream experiences.

- **Improve Dream Recall:** Sometimes, you may become lucid but forget the experience upon waking. Improving your dream recall (through dream journaling and intention setting) will help you recognize more lucid dreams.

2. Losing Lucidity
Another common issue is losing lucidity once it's achieved. You may become lucid for a brief moment, only to slip back into a regular dream.
Here's how to maintain lucidity:

- **Stay Calm:** Excitement can quickly cause you to wake up or lose focus in a dream. When you first realize you're dreaming, take a moment to calm yourself. Focus on your surroundings and use grounding techniques (e.g., rubbing your hands together or touching objects in the dream) to stabilize the dream.

- **Engage the Dream World:** One reason people lose lucidity is because they become passive within the dream. Once you're lucid, actively engage with the dream world—ask questions, interact with dream characters, or explore the environment.

Staying mentally engaged helps you maintain lucidity.

- **Remind Yourself:** Periodically remind yourself that you're dreaming. This will help reinforce your lucidity and prevent you from slipping back into a non-lucid state.

3. Waking Up Too Early
It's common for beginners to wake up too soon after becoming lucid, either from excitement or because the dream begins to destabilize. Here's how to prolong your lucid dreams:

- **Dream Stabilization Techniques:** If you feel the dream fading, try focusing on the sensory aspects of the dream to ground yourself in the experience. Spin around in the dream, rub your hands together, or touch objects to engage your senses. This helps anchor you in the dream and prevents early wake-ups.

- **Don't Focus on Your Body:** Thinking about your physical body (lying in bed) while in a dream can cause you to wake up. Keep your focus on the dream world and avoid thinking about waking life.

4. Difficulty Controlling the Dream
While becoming lucid is the first step, learning how to control the dream can be challenging. Some dreamers struggle to influence the environment or manipulate the dream as they desire. Here are some strategies:

- **Start Small:** If you're having trouble controlling large aspects of the dream, start with small changes. For example, try changing the color of an object or levitating slightly above the ground. Once you gain confidence, you can move on to larger tasks like flying or creating entire dream scenes.

- **Use Commands:** In the dream, use verbal commands to influence the environment. For example, if you want to fly, say, "Fly!" aloud, and imagine the sensation of lifting off the ground. Verbal commands can help direct your subconscious mind to follow your desires.

- **Believe in Your Control:** In lucid dreams, your expectations often dictate what happens. If you doubt your ability to control the dream, you're less likely to succeed. Approach dream control with confidence and an open mind, trusting that you have the power to shape the dream.

5. False Awakenings

A false awakening is when you "wake up" from a dream, only to realize later that you were still dreaming. These can be disorienting and frustrating, especially if you lose lucidity. Here's how to handle false awakenings:

- Perform a Reality Check: Whenever you wake up, get into the habit of performing a reality check right away.

False awakenings are often very realistic, but a quick check (such as the nose pinch test) can reveal that you're still dreaming.

- **Stay Aware After Becoming Lucid:** Once you've become lucid, remind yourself to stay alert, especially when transitioning between dream scenes. This will help you avoid false awakenings and maintain lucidity.

By addressing these challenges and refining your techniques, you can improve your lucid dreaming practice and achieve more consistent, controlled, and fulfilling experiences.

A Guide to Dream Control

Once you've achieved lucidity, the dream world opens up like an unexplored universe, filled with endless possibilities. But becoming lucid is only the first step; the real adventure begins when you learn how to control and shape your dreams. Dream control can be both thrilling and challenging. It requires not only an understanding of how dreams work but also a level of mental flexibility and belief in your ability to manipulate the environment around you. In this chapter, we'll dive into various techniques for controlling your dreams, exploring the many ways you can experiment with the dream world. When you first achieve lucidity, your instinct may be to immediately start controlling everything around you—

flying, conjuring people or objects, or changing the dream's entire landscape. However, for beginners, maintaining control can be difficult, especially if the excitement of realizing you're dreaming makes the dream unstable. One of the first things you'll need to practice is staying calm.

Excitement is natural, but it can be disruptive. A useful grounding technique is to pause as soon as you become lucid and focus on your dream environment. Try to touch something, like a wall or an object, and really feel its texture. Engage your senses—this will help stabilize the dream and ground you in it.

Once you've stabilized the dream, you can start experimenting with smaller acts of control. In many cases, manipulating the dream requires you to truly believe in the malleability of the dream world. If you doubt your ability to fly or transform the scenery, the dream might resist your attempts.

This is because dreams are often shaped by your subconscious expectations. For instance, if you're trying to fly but find yourself hovering close to the ground, your subconscious may be doubting that flying is possible. The key is to let go of those doubts and focus on the sensation of what you want to achieve.

A helpful way to take control of your dreams is to start by interacting with the elements that already exist in the dream. For example, if you find yourself in a familiar place, like your childhood home, try altering small aspects of it. Change the color of the walls or transform an everyday object into something unusual, like turning a chair into a tree. Starting with small changes builds your confidence and gradually allows you to take on more ambitious acts of dream control.

Flying is one of the most common goals for lucid dreamers, and there are several methods to achieve it. Some dreamers find success by simply imagining themselves taking off the ground, while others use a tool within the dream—such as a vehicle or even wings—to help them get airborne.

f you find yourself struggling to fly, try taking a leap and allowing gravity to let go. The sensation of lifting off will often trigger the freedom to fly. Another method is to imagine a strong wind or force lifting you up. Remember, the key to controlling your dream is belief. If you believe you can fly, you will.

Another exciting aspect of lucid dreaming is interacting with dream characters. These characters can be manifestations of people from your real life, fictional creations, or sometimes completely unknown figures. Many lucid dreamers use their dreams to speak to these characters in search of insight or simply for the experience of interacting with their subconscious.

Dream characters can behave in unexpected ways, sometimes offering profound insights or responding with strange, nonsensical answers. As you gain more experience in lucid dreaming, you can experiment with summoning specific characters, whether they are real people or entirely imaginary beings.

One of the most intriguing abilities in lucid dreaming is the power to create entirely new dream environments. This is where the dream truly becomes your personal playground. You can teleport from one place to another simply by imagining yourself in a different location. Some dreamers visualize a door, and when they open it, they step into a completely new world. Others find success by spinning around quickly in the dream, which causes the scenery to blur and shift into something new when they stop. You can visit fantastical worlds, recreate places from your past, or design entirely new landscapes. The limits of dream creation are bound only by your imagination.

At some point, you may encounter resistance in your dreams—perhaps you try to change something and find that the dream resists your control.

This resistance usually stems from the subconscious mind, which can sometimes interfere with your conscious intentions. When this happens, it's important to remain patient and not force control.

Instead, take a step back and try engaging with the dream in a different way. For instance, if you can't change a dream character's appearance or behavior, try speaking to them and asking why they are acting a certain way.

Often, your subconscious will provide an answer, and from there, you can work with the dream rather than against it.

Finally, dream stabilization techniques are crucial for maintaining control, especially if you feel the dream slipping away. Dream spinning is one such technique—when the dream begins to fade or blur, spin your body around in circles within the dream.

The sensation of spinning will engage your senses and pull you deeper into the dream, often causing the environment to reset or stabilize. Similarly, rubbing your hands together creates a tactile sensation that can help ground you in the dream world, preventing you from waking up prematurely.

Mastering dream control takes time, but it's a deeply rewarding process. As you gain more experience, you'll discover just how versatile and creative your dreams can be. Whether you're flying through the sky, exploring distant planets, or creating entire cities with your mind, dream control allows you to tap into the limitless potential of your subconscious.

Advanced Techniques: Layering and Stabilization

As you become more proficient at lucid dreaming, you can begin to explore advanced techniques that allow for deeper control and richer experiences. One such technique is **dream layering**, where you enter multiple lucid dreams within a single sleep cycle. Another key skill is **stabilization**, which helps prevent dreams from collapsing or fading too quickly. Mastering these advanced techniques can lead to more vivid, extended, and satisfying lucid dreams.

Dream layering involves transitioning from one lucid dream to another while maintaining awareness. It's a phenomenon where you "wake up" within a dream, only to realize that you're still dreaming. This can occur naturally, especially when you have a **false awakening** (when you dream that you've woken up but are still in a dream). With practice, you can learn to control this process and deliberately enter new dream layers.

Layering begins when you recognize that you're in a lucid dream and choose to leave that dream to enter another one. Some dreamers use the false awakening technique to move into the next layer. If you realize you've had a false awakening—such as waking up in your bedroom only to discover that it's still a dream—you can use this opportunity to deepen your lucid state. The key to dream layering is remaining calm and maintaining your lucidity during the transition between layers. You might find that each subsequent dream layer feels more vivid or that your level of control increases as you go deeper.

Layering can also be triggered intentionally by using visualization. If you want to enter a new dream layer, imagine yourself "falling asleep" within the dream. This mental shift often brings you into a new, deeper dream environment. However, there is a caveat—going too deep into dream layers can sometimes make it harder to maintain lucidity, especially for beginners. For this reason, it's essential to stabilize each dream layer before attempting to transition to the next.

Stabilization is one of the most critical skills for any lucid dreamer, especially when dreams start to become unstable or fragment. Lucid dreams, particularly for beginners, can often feel fragile, with scenes shifting rapidly or dream characters fading away unexpectedly. When this happens, it's vital to have techniques ready to anchor yourself more firmly in the dream world.

One of the most effective stabilization techniques is **engaging your senses**. Focusing on tactile sensations, such as feeling the texture of objects in your dream or rubbing your hands together, helps reinforce the reality of the dream. Touch is particularly effective because it forces your mind to concentrate on the physical aspects of the dream, grounding your awareness.

Another powerful stabilization method is **dream spinning**. When you feel a dream starting to dissolve, spinning around within the dream can reset the environment, helping you regain control. As you spin, the motion distracts your mind from the destabilization, allowing the dream to reform around you. Spinning also engages your sense of motion, which can help anchor you in the dream.

Verbal commands can also be useful for stabilizing a dream. If you feel the dream starting to fade, saying phrases like "Stay focused" or "Stabilize" aloud within the dream can reinforce your intention to remain lucid. These commands send a clear signal to your subconscious mind that you want to maintain the dream.

Visual focus is another technique for stabilization. When dreams start to blur or lose detail, focusing on a single object—whether it's your hands, a piece of furniture, or a part of the dream landscape—can help bring clarity back to the dream. By zeroing in on one detail, you encourage your mind to reengage with the dream's environment, preventing it from collapsing.

Dream stabilization isn't just about keeping a dream from ending prematurely—it's also about deepening the dream experience. The more stable the dream, the more vivid and immersive it becomes. With practice, you'll find that stabilization becomes second nature, allowing you to maintain lucidity for extended periods and explore dreams more fully.

Mastering these advanced techniques will take your lucid dreaming practice to a new level, offering greater control, longer dream experiences, and more profound insights into the workings of your subconscious mind.

Lucid Dreaming for Problem-Solving

One of the most powerful applications of lucid dreaming is its potential to enhance creativity and solve problems. In the dream state, the mind operates without the constraints of waking logic, allowing ideas to flow freely and offering new perspectives on challenges you face in waking life. Many famous artists, writers, and inventors have used dreams—lucid or otherwise—as a source of inspiration and innovation.

The dream world is an ideal environment for creative exploration because it operates on the same principles as imagination, but in a more vivid and immersive way. When you're lucid, you can deliberately tap into this wellspring of creativity by setting specific goals for your dreams. For example, if you're a writer, you can use a lucid dream to explore new plot ideas, experiment with different characters, or even see a story unfold visually in front of you. Similarly, artists can use their dreams to visualize new concepts, play with abstract forms, or discover new color schemes that they might not have thought of in their waking state.

Many famous creative minds have credited their dreams with inspiring breakthroughs. Salvador Dalí, the renowned surrealist painter, often used his dreams as the basis for his fantastical, dream-like artwork. He even developed techniques to induce dream-like states, such as holding a spoon over a plate while falling asleep, so the sound of the spoon dropping would wake him at the perfect moment between wakefulness and dreaming— allowing him to capture the surreal imagery his subconscious produced.

Lucid dreaming takes this creative exploration a step further by giving you active control over the dream. Instead of passively experiencing a dream's narrative, you can direct it toward specific goals. If you're trying to solve a creative problem—whether it's finishing a novel, composing music, or designing something—you can consciously ask your dream to show you a solution. Because dreams draw from the vast resources of your subconscious, they often provide surprising and innovative answers that your waking mind might not have considered.

Lucid dreaming is also a powerful tool for problem-solving in a more practical sense. The brain's ability to think laterally in a dream allows for creative problem-solving that often feels elusive during waking life. Many people have reported waking up with solutions to complex problems after dreaming about them. This is because, in dreams, the subconscious mind processes information differently. It's not bound by the constraints of logic, which means it can approach problems from unique angles.

For instance, if you're working on a difficult project at work or school, you can bring the problem into your lucid dream. Set the intention before going to sleep that you want to find a solution to the problem. Once you're lucid, you can interact with your dream environment or ask dream characters for advice. Often, the subconscious will present creative solutions that hadn't occurred to you while awake.

You can also use lucid dreaming as a space to rehearse scenarios and practice new skills. Because the dream world mimics reality in many ways, it provides a safe environment to experiment with new ideas or refine skills. For example, if you're preparing for a public presentation, you can practice delivering your speech in a lucid dream. The heightened realism of the dream will make the practice feel authentic, helping you build confidence and refine your delivery for when you face the real-life scenario.

Lucid dreaming also allows for the resolution of personal conflicts or emotional dilemmas. If you're facing a difficult decision or struggling with a relationship issue, you can explore different outcomes in your dream, allowing you to see the situation from multiple perspectives. Dream characters can act as stand-ins for people in your waking life, enabling you to have conversations or confrontations that you might avoid while awake. By resolving conflicts in the dream, you often gain clarity and insight that helps in real life.

As you continue to practice lucid dreaming, you'll discover that the dream world is not just a place for personal exploration and enjoyment—it's a powerful tool for tapping into your deepest creative potential and solving real-world problems. Whether you're looking to unlock a new creative idea or find a solution to a difficult challenge, lucid dreaming offers a unique and profound way to access the hidden resources of your mind.

Lucid Dreaming and Out-of-Body Experiences: The Difference

Lucid dreaming and out-of-body experiences (OBEs) are often confused with one another, as both involve altered states of consciousness that allow the individual to perceive themselves outside of their normal waking reality. However, they are distinct phenomena, each with its own characteristics, methods of induction, and subjective experiences.

Understanding the differences between the two can help you navigate these experiences more effectively and use them for your personal growth.

Lucid dreaming occurs within the context of sleep, specifically during REM sleep when vivid dreams are most likely to occur. In a lucid dream, you become aware that you are dreaming and can then take control of the dream environment, interacting with it consciously.

The hallmark of lucid dreaming is that it takes place within the mind, and while the dream feels real, you know that your physical body is asleep in bed.

In contrast, an out-of-body experience typically occurs when you feel that your consciousness has left your physical body and is existing independently of it. OBEs can occur in various states, including sleep, near-death experiences, or even during deep meditation.

People who experience OBEs often report floating above their physical body, seeing themselves from a third-person perspective, and exploring their environment in a disembodied state. Unlike lucid dreaming, OBEs often feel more "real" and less dream-like, with individuals describing a heightened sense of awareness and clarity.

One of the main differences between the two experiences lies in how they are induced. Lucid dreams usually occur spontaneously, although they can be intentionally triggered using techniques such as reality checks or the Wake-Induced Lucid Dreaming (WILD) method. OBEs, on the other hand, often happen during states of extreme relaxation, such as deep meditation or when the body is on the verge of sleep but the mind remains awake. OBEs can also be induced deliberately through techniques like **astral projection**, where the individual uses visualization and relaxation methods to separate their consciousness from their body.

While both lucid dreaming and OBEs involve a sense of freedom and detachment from the physical body, the nature of the experience differs. In a lucid dream, the environment is typically malleable and shaped by your subconscious thoughts and desires.

You can change the scenery, interact with dream characters, and experience fantastical scenarios that defy the laws of physics.

In an OBE, however, the environment is usually perceived as more static and grounded in reality. People who have OBEs often report traveling to familiar locations or observing their physical surroundings in great detail. Another key difference is the level of control you have in each experience. In a lucid dream, you can exert a high degree of control over the dream world, making things appear or disappear, flying through the air, or manipulating the narrative. In an OBE, the experience is often more passive, with the individual simply observing their surroundings rather than actively controlling them. However, advanced OBE practitioners can learn to navigate different planes of existence, traveling beyond the physical world into what is sometimes described as the astral plane.

For those interested in exploring both lucid dreaming and OBEs, it's important to recognize that the skills used to induce these experiences are similar. Practices such as mindfulness, relaxation, and visualization can help you achieve both states. However, the intentions and outcomes of these experiences may vary. Some people use lucid dreaming as a tool for creativity, self-exploration, or personal enjoyment, while OBEs are often associated with spiritual exploration or a desire to connect with a higher state of consciousness.

Ultimately, both lucid dreaming and out-of-body experiences offer valuable insights into the nature of consciousness and the mind's ability to transcend ordinary reality. Whether you're looking to control your dreams or explore the boundaries of your awareness, these experiences provide a fascinating window into the limitless potential of the human mind.

Healing and Self-Transformation through Lucid Dreaming

Lucid dreaming is not only a tool for exploration and creativity; it can also be a profound method for emotional healing and personal transformation. By engaging with your dreams consciously, you can unlock hidden emotions, work through past traumas, and reframe your experiences in ways that promote healing and growth. In this chapter, we will explore how you can use lucid dreams to heal emotional wounds and transform your inner self.

Dreams are often a reflection of our subconscious minds, where unprocessed emotions and unresolved conflicts reside. During regular dreams, these issues may appear symbolically—perhaps in the form of distressing scenarios or recurring nightmares. In a lucid dream, however, you have the unique opportunity to confront these issues directly, making it possible to reshape the narrative and change how you experience them.

One of the most powerful ways to initiate healing in a lucid dream is by intentionally facing your fears. For example, if you frequently have nightmares about being chased, becoming lucid in the dream allows you to stop running and confront the pursuer. You can ask the dream figure what they represent or what message they have for you.

This dialogue often reveals deeper emotional truths or insights into unresolved issues from your waking life. Once you understand the symbolism behind the fear, you can transform it, either by neutralizing the threat or changing the dream's outcome to something more positive.

Lucid dreaming can also be a therapeutic space for processing grief and loss. Some people use lucid dreams to reconnect with loved ones who have passed away, giving them a sense of closure or an opportunity to express emotions they couldn't in waking life. While the dream characters aren't literal representations of those individuals, they often embody the dreamer's emotional experiences, providing a meaningful way to process unresolved feelings.

Self-compassion is another area where lucid dreaming can be transformative.

In a lucid dream, you can engage in self-dialogue, either by speaking to a version of yourself within the dream or by guiding the dream narrative to focus on self-care and healing. Imagine yourself in a comforting environment—such as a peaceful forest or beside a warm fire—and allow your subconscious mind to bring forth whatever emotions need to be addressed.

By offering kindness and compassion to yourself in the dream, you can foster a deeper sense of self-acceptance and emotional healing that extends into your waking life. Lucid dreaming also offers an opportunity for personal transformation by enabling you to rehearse new behaviors or break free from limiting beliefs.

If you struggle with self-confidence or anxiety in certain situations, you can use your lucid dreams as a safe space to practice responding differently.

For example, if public speaking makes you nervous, you can create a dream scenario where you're delivering a speech to a large audience. Because the dream feels real, the practice you gain carries over into waking life, helping to reduce anxiety and build confidence.

By consciously engaging with the emotional and symbolic content of your dreams, you can initiate powerful changes within yourself. The insights and healing you experience in lucid dreams can lead to profound personal transformation, allowing you to overcome past wounds, strengthen your sense of self, and develop a deeper understanding of your inner world.

.

The Spiritual Dimensions of Lucid Dreaming

For many people, lucid dreaming isn't just a psychological or creative practice—it is also a deeply spiritual experience. Throughout history, various cultures and spiritual traditions have viewed dreams as a gateway to higher states of consciousness, and lucid dreaming has often been used as a tool for spiritual growth and enlightenment.

In this chapter, we will explore the spiritual dimensions of lucid dreaming, including its connections to meditation, mindfulness, and the exploration of consciousness.

In Tibetan Buddhism, there is a practice known as **dream yoga**, which is considered one of the six yogas of Naropa, designed to bring practitioners closer to enlightenment. Dream yoga involves becoming conscious in the dream state and using that awareness to recognize the illusory nature of all experiences, both waking and dreaming. By cultivating lucidity in dreams, practitioners learn to dissolve attachments and fears, leading to a deeper understanding of the true nature of reality.

Dream yoga teaches that life itself is much like a dream—fleeting and impermanent.

Through this practice, individuals can develop spiritual insight, freeing themselves from the delusions of the material world.

Lucid dreaming also provides a unique opportunity for deepening mindfulness and meditation practices. In a lucid dream, the heightened awareness and control allow you to engage in meditative practices, such as focusing on the breath or visualizing spiritual symbols. Because the dream state is highly immersive, these meditations can be incredibly vivid, often leading to profound insights or mystical experiences.

Some lucid dreamers report achieving states of pure awareness, where they feel connected to a universal consciousness or experience a sense of transcendence beyond the physical world.

Another spiritual aspect of lucid dreaming is the exploration of **the astral plane**, a concept found in various mystical traditions. In this context, the astral plane is thought to be a non-physical dimension where consciousness exists independent of the body.

Some people believe that lucid dreaming can be used as a gateway to this plane, allowing dreamers to explore spiritual realms and interact with higher beings or spiritual guides. While the existence of the astral plane is a matter of belief, many lucid dreamers describe their experiences in these realms as deeply spiritual and transformative.

Lucid dreaming can also be used as a tool for exploring the concept of **life after death**. Some people believe that the dream state offers a glimpse into what happens to consciousness after the body dies, with lucid dreaming serving as a way to explore the nature of the soul and its connection to the universe.

Whether or not you believe in these spiritual interpretations, lucid dreams can provide profound experiences that challenge your understanding of reality, consciousness, and existence itself.

For those on a spiritual path, lucid dreaming offers a powerful way to deepen their practice and connect with their higher self. Whether you use your lucid dreams to meditate, explore mystical realms, or seek guidance from your subconscious, the dream state provides a unique and expansive space for spiritual exploration.

Lucid Dreaming and Creativity in the Arts

Lucid dreaming has long been recognized as a powerful tool for artists, musicians, writers, and other creatives. The dream world offers an endless canvas for the imagination, where the normal constraints of time, space, and logic do not apply. In this chapter, we will explore how lucid dreaming can be harnessed to enhance creativity in the arts, providing real-world examples of how famous artists have used their dreams to inspire groundbreaking work.

The creative potential of lucid dreams is vast because dreams naturally tap into the subconscious mind, where ideas, memories, and emotions mingle freely. For artists, this unbounded space can lead to unique insights and fresh perspectives. When lucid, the dreamer has the ability to interact with these subconscious elements in a conscious way, which makes it possible to experiment with new artistic techniques, visualize complex compositions, or explore entirely new creative concepts.

One of the most famous examples of lucid dreaming in the arts comes from the surrealist painter **Salvador Dalí**, who used his dreams as a source of inspiration for much of his work. Dalí is known for his dream-like imagery, full of melting clocks, floating objects, and other surreal distortions of reality.

He developed techniques for inducing dream-like states while awake, but he also drew extensively from his lucid dreams, where he would actively explore bizarre and surreal landscapes. By bridging the gap between his waking and dreaming worlds, Dalí was able to create some of the most iconic and imaginative works of the 20th century.

In literature, dreams have long been a source of inspiration. **Mary Shelley**, the author of *Frankenstein*, famously credited a dream with sparking the idea for her groundbreaking novel. In her dream, she envisioned a scientist bringing a corpse to life through a mysterious process, a vision that became the foundation for her story. Similarly, **Robert Louis Stevenson**, the author of *The Strange Case of Dr. Jekyll and Mr. Hyde*, reported that two of the novel's key scenes came to him in a dream, providing the inspiration he needed to complete the story. Lucid dreaming allows creatives to go a step further by giving them direct control over their dream environments. If you are a visual artist, you can use your lucid dreams to experiment with colors, shapes, and textures in ways that are impossible in waking life. If you are a musician, you can compose melodies or rhythms that emerge organically from your subconscious. Writers can explore entire narratives in their dreams, observing characters and plotlines unfold in real-time.

Beyond direct inspiration, lucid dreaming can also be a space for solving creative blocks. If you're stuck on a project or struggling with an idea, you can set an intention before going to sleep to work through the problem in your dream. Once you become lucid, you can ask for guidance from a dream character, explore different scenarios, or simply allow your mind to play with the issue in a more fluid, relaxed way. Many lucid dreamers find that when they wake up, they have new insights or solutions that weren't apparent while they were awake.

For anyone involved in the arts, lucid dreaming offers an unparalleled tool for exploring creativity, breaking through mental barriers, and discovering new ways of expressing themselves. The dream world is limitless, and for artists, it provides a wellspring of inspiration that can fuel their work for years to come.

The Ethics and Responsibilities of Lucid Dreaming

While lucid dreaming can be a powerful tool for exploration and personal growth, it also comes with certain ethical considerations. As with any practice that involves deep self-exploration, there are potential risks and responsibilities that come with lucid dreaming, particularly when it comes to how we interact with the dream world and the people within it.

In this chapter, we will explore the ethics of lucid dreaming, including the potential psychological effects and the responsibilities dreamers have to themselves and others.

One ethical consideration involves the treatment of dream characters. In a lucid dream, the characters you encounter may appear as independent beings, but they are often reflections of your own subconscious mind. Some dreamers may be tempted to manipulate or control these characters in ways that could be considered unethical, even if they are only figments of the dream world.

For instance, using lucid dreams to harm or dominate dream characters could lead to negative psychological consequences, reinforcing harmful behaviors or attitudes that might carry over into waking life.

There is also the question of consent within dreams. If you use your dreams to interact with real-life people, it's important to remember that while these characters are not the actual individuals, they represent your perceptions of them.

Treating dream versions of people with respect and empathy can help reinforce positive relationships in waking life. On the other hand, using your dreams to manipulate or mistreat others—even in a subconscious form—could reflect unresolved issues or unhealthy attitudes that need to be addressed.

Lucid dreaming also requires a certain level of responsibility in how it is integrated into daily life. While the dream world offers freedom and escapism, it's important not to become overly dependent on it as a way of avoiding real-world challenges. Lucid dreaming should be used as a tool for growth, self-exploration, and creativity, not as an escape from reality.

For individuals prone to dissociation or mental health issues, there is a potential risk of becoming too attached to the dream world, which can blur the boundaries between dreaming and waking life. In these cases, it's important to approach lucid dreaming with caution and, if necessary, seek guidance from a mental health professional.

Another ethical consideration is the use of lucid dreaming for personal gain.

While it's tempting to use lucid dreams to rehearse real-life situations for personal advantage—such as practicing negotiations, interviews, or interactions with others—it's important to remain mindful of the potential consequences.

Using dreams to gain an edge in waking life can be beneficial when done with integrity, but it's crucial to ensure that this advantage does not come at the expense of honesty or fairness.

Finally, lucid dreaming also opens up philosophical questions about the nature of reality and consciousness. If we can control our dream worlds, how does this impact our understanding of free will, agency, and the self?

For some, lucid dreaming raises ethical questions about the nature of consciousness itself—what responsibilities do we have, not just to our waking selves, but to the dream world we create and inhabit?

In navigating these ethical dilemmas, it's important to approach lucid dreaming with a sense of curiosity, compassion, and responsibility. By treating the dream world and its inhabitants with the same respect you would in waking life, you can ensure that your lucid dreaming practice remains a positive, enriching experience that contributes to your personal growth and well-being.

Final Thoughts on Lucid Dreaming

As we conclude this journey into the fascinating world of lucid dreaming, it's essential to take a moment to reflect on everything you've learned and experienced. Lucid dreaming is more than just a tool for creative exploration, personal enjoyment, or problem-solving—it's a gateway into the deepest recesses of your mind and, more profoundly, into the nature of your consciousness. The journey toward mastering lucid dreaming is, in many ways, a journey toward mastering your own inner landscape, and, by extension, your life.

Lucid dreaming has taught you how to navigate your dreams with intention and awareness, but its lessons extend far beyond the dream state.

The skills you've developed—mindfulness, focus, imagination, and emotional intelligence—are the same skills that enhance your waking life.

Lucid dreaming offers a unique perspective, reminding us that the boundaries of reality are more fluid than we might believe. It challenges the rigid structures of logic and linearity that govern our waking lives and invites us to explore the vast possibilities that exist within the mind. At the heart of lucid dreaming is the idea that you can shape your reality.

In dreams, you are the creator of worlds. You have the power to fly, to meet anyone you wish, to visit any place, and to experience anything that your imagination can conjure.

This power, however, is not limited to dreams. In many ways, the lessons of lucid dreaming apply directly to how we shape our waking realities.

When you learn to recognize and change limiting beliefs in your dreams, you begin to realize that similar limitations often exist in waking life—beliefs that hold you back, fears that keep you grounded, and mental habits that stifle your creativity.

Lucid dreaming teaches you that with awareness and intention, you can break through these barriers, both in your dreams and in your daily life.

Consider the implications of what you've learned. In your dreams, you've faced fears head-on, transformed nightmares into empowering experiences, and embraced the impossible with confidence and joy.

These achievements are not confined to the dream world; they are reflections of your mind's potential.

When you confront a fear in a dream—perhaps by turning to face a pursuer or resolving a deep-seated emotional issue—you're practicing the art of confronting fear in waking life.

This is one of the most profound benefits of lucid dreaming: the ability to transcend fear, not just in the safety of the dream but in your everyday experiences. For those who have delved into the spiritual dimensions of lucid dreaming, the practice offers even deeper insights. Lucid dreaming can lead to experiences that transcend the individual self, providing a sense of connection to something greater—whether you frame it as a universal consciousness, the divine, or simply a heightened state of awareness.

The ability to recognize the dream state is, in many ways, a metaphor for waking up to the deeper truths of existence. When you learn to see through the illusions of the dream, you're also practicing the ability to see through the illusions of everyday life—the judgments, attachments, and fears that keep you from experiencing life fully.

The dream world is not just an escape or an alternate reality; it's a reflection of your innermost thoughts, desires, and emotions.

As you've progressed in your practice, you've likely noticed recurring themes, patterns, and symbols that appear in your dreams. These are direct expressions of your subconscious mind, and they offer valuable insights into your waking self.

When you dream of flying, for instance, you might be tapping into a desire for freedom or transcendence. When you encounter a recurring dream figure, you may be engaging with an aspect of yourself that you have yet to fully understand.

Lucid dreaming provides the unique opportunity to engage with these symbols consciously, allowing you to learn more about yourself and, in doing so, integrate different aspects of your psyche into a more unified whole.

In your lucid dreaming journey, you may have also discovered that dreams have their own logic and rules, which sometimes resist your control.

This teaches an important lesson: while you can shape your experiences, both in dreams and in life, there will always be elements beyond your control. This is part of the mystery and beauty of life itself.

Lucid dreaming reminds us that, while we have immense creative power, true mastery comes not from controlling every detail but from learning to flow with the dream— trusting the process, adapting to changes, and allowing the dream (and life) to unfold as it will.

This balance between intention and acceptance is a key lesson not just for lucid dreaming but for living a fulfilling and harmonious life.

Lucid dreaming also teaches the importance of patience and persistence. If you're like most dreamers, you didn't achieve lucidity overnight.

t took practice—whether through keeping a dream journal, performing reality checks, or mastering advanced techniques like WILD or MILD.

There were likely moments of frustration, when dreams slipped away before you could gain control or when lucidity felt just out of reach.

But with each attempt, you learned something new, whether it was a deeper understanding of your sleep cycles or a better technique for stabilizing a dream.

In this way, lucid dreaming mirrors the learning process in all areas of life. Success comes from dedication, from showing up consistently, even when progress seems slow. The rewards, however, are immense—whether it's the thrill of flying through a dreamscape or the quiet satisfaction of mastering a new skill.

Now that you've gained a deeper understanding of lucid dreaming, the question becomes: how will you continue to use this practice in your life?

For many, lucid dreaming is not just a fleeting interest but a lifelong pursuit, a continual exploration of the mind's infinite possibilities.

Some dreamers may choose to focus on creativity, using lucid dreams as a space to experiment with artistic ideas, solve problems, or explore new worlds. Others may delve into the therapeutic potential of dreams, using them to process emotions, resolve internal conflicts, and foster emotional healing. Still others may pursue lucid dreaming as a spiritual practice, seeking greater awareness and enlightenment through the dream state.

Whatever path you choose, remember that the journey of lucid dreaming is an ongoing one.

Just as your dreams evolve, so too will your relationship with them. There will always be new techniques to learn, new challenges to face, and new experiences to enjoy. Lucid dreaming is a dynamic practice, one that grows with you as you grow.

As you deepen your practice, you'll find that the boundaries between waking life and dream life begin to blur.

The skills you develop in your dreams—such as mindfulness, creativity, and emotional resilience—will enhance your waking experiences, just as your waking life will influence the content of your dreams.

In the end, lucid dreaming offers a powerful reminder that life itself is a creative act. Just as you shape your dreams, you have the power to shape your reality. Your thoughts, beliefs, and intentions are the tools with which you create your world—both in sleep and in waking life. Lucid dreaming invites you to embrace this creative potential fully, to live with greater intention, awareness, and joy. Whether you're soaring through the skies of your dreams or navigating the challenges of daily life, remember that you are the creator of your experience.

As you close this book and continue your journey, take with you the knowledge that lucid dreaming is not just a skill—it is a way of thinking, a way of being.

It teaches you to wake up, not only in your dreams but in your life. To be aware, to be present, and to embrace the extraordinary potential within you.

The journey of lucid dreaming doesn't end when you wake up.

It continues in every moment of your waking life, as you carry the lessons, insights, and experiences from your dreams into your daily reality. Whether you're just beginning your exploration of lucid dreaming or are already an experienced dreamer, the possibilities are limitless. Your dreams are a canvas, and with lucidity, you hold the brush.

Thank you for embarking on this journey into the world of lucid dreaming.

May your dreams be filled with wonder, insight, and infinite possibilities, and may your waking life be just as vivid, creative, and intentional as the worlds you create in your sleep.

This is just the beginning of your lucid journey—your dreams await.

Disclaimer

The implementation of all information, instructions and strategies contained in this book is at your own risk. The author cannot accept liability for any damages of any kind on any legal grounds. Liability claims against the author for material or immaterial damage caused by the use or non-use of the information or by the use of incorrect and/or incomplete information are fundamentally excluded. Any legal claims and claims for damages are therefore also excluded. This work has been compiled and written down with the utmost care and to the best of our knowledge and belief. However, the author accepts no liability for the topicality, completeness and quality of the information. Printing errors and incorrect information cannot be completely ruled out. No legal responsibility or liability of any kind can be accepted for incorrect information provided by the author.

Copyright

All contents of this work as well as information, strategies and tips are protected by copyright. All rights reserved. Any reprinting or reproduction - even in part - in any form such as photocopying or similar processes, storage, processing, duplication and distribution by means of electronic systems of any kind (in whole or in part) is strictly prohibited without the express written permission of the author. All translation rights reserved. The contents may not be published under any circumstances. The author reserves the right to take legal action in the event of non-compliance.

Imprint

Made in United States
Troutdale, OR
10/26/2024

24145395R00046